You've Got This! Companion Workbook

Published by:
Soaring Seagull Press
Santa Rosa, CA 95401
EatingFor.com

© 2023 Soaring Seagull Press. All rights reserved.

No part of this book, including interior design, cover design and illustrations may be reproduced, stored in a retrieval system or transmitted by any means, electronic, mechanical, photocopying, recording or otherwise, without written permission from the authors and publisher, except for the inclusion of brief quotations in a review.

Although every precaution has been taken in the preparation of this book, the authors and publisher assume no responsibility for errors or omissions. The authors and publisher expressly disclaim any responsibility for any liability, loss, injury or risk, personal or otherwise, which is incurred as a consequence, directly or indirectly, of the use and application of any of the contents of this book.

The information in this book is provided for educational purposes and general reference. It is not meant to be a substitute for medical advice or counseling. Consult a physician before making any changes to diet, exercise or other health habits as described in this book.

ISBN: 978-0-9848540-2-8

Printed in the United States of America

Instructions

While this workbook is designed to be a companion to *You've Got This! 45 Doable Tips for Teens to Feel Good, Look Good & Succeed*, it can do double duty as a standalone workbook for teens and young adults alike who want to set and track any goal that matters. Here's how it works:

1. Choose

Each week, write down a goal you want to achieve. If you're feeling motivated, write down two or three. Be sure to make them SMART goals so they're easier to track. (You'll find all the details on the next page.)

2. Doodle, Dream & Do

Doodle, dream and write down your thoughts every day so you can get your creative juices flowing, activate deep learning and let the problem solving begin.

3. Review

Review your progress every day and celebrate your wins, especially the small changes that move the dial toward ultimate success. After all, these small changes are the real secret behind shaping success habits that last a lifetime.

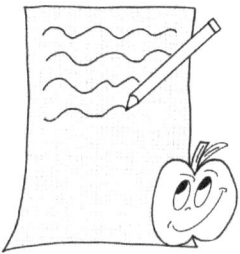

SMART Goals

SMART stands for the five key elements of an effective goal: **S**pecific, **M**easurable, **A**ttainable, **R**ealistic and **T**imed. For example, the goal "I will drink 8 cups of water every day this week" is a SMART goal. Here's why:

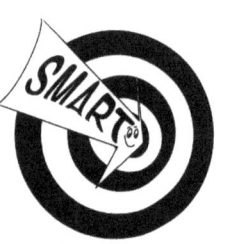

S   **Specific.** The goal aims to drink more water (rather than just beverages).

M   **Measurable.** The goal aims to drink 8 cups of water per day (rather than just drink more water).

A   **Attainable.** The goal is attainable because water is readily available.

R   **Realistic.** The goal is neither too difficult (which can be frustrating), nor too easy (which can lead to boredom).

T   **Time sensitive.** The goal has a deadline (one week), so you can measure your progress, see what's working and what may need adjusting.

You can apply the SMART approach to any goal that matters. To get started, check out the example on the next page.

Do's

WEEK OF _____

GOALS FOR THIS WEEK
① 8 cups of water each day.
② 2 vegetables at dinner.
③ Walk 10,000 steps each day.

MONDAY ✓✓✓
Easier to drink more water with lemon. A lot of steamed carrots and broccoli today, need to mix it up more.

TUESDAY ✓✓✓
3-bean soup really helped me up the variety of veggies today.

WEDNESDAY ✓✓
What a busy day! Water intake good, veggies good, but didn't get my steps in. Tomorrow will be better.

THURSDAY ✓✓✓
11,200 steps today. Using a phone app to track steps really helps. Great day!

FRIDAY ✓✓✓
Dinner out. So proud of myself for ordering a steamed veggie rice bowl.

SATURDAY ✓✓✓
Bringing a water bottle with me really helps me drink more. Need to make this a habit.

SUNDAY ✓✓✓
Tried Portobello mushrooms over mashed potatoes for the first time. Yum. Feeling great about this week's progress. ☺

The two most important days in your life are the day you are born and the day you find out why.
— Mark Twain

Doodles & Dreams

FEEL GOOD Tip #1 For good grades and an active social life, turn to the power of sleep.

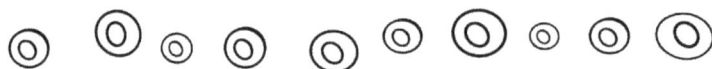

Do'y

Week of _____

Goals for this week
① _____
② _____
③ _____

Monday ① ② ③

Tuesday ① ② ③

Wednesday ① ② ③

Thursday ① ② ③

Friday ① ② ③

Saturday ① ② ③

Sunday ① ② ③

A journey of a thousand miles begins with a single step.
—*Lao Tzu*

Doodles & Dreams

FEEL GOOD Tip #2 For peak performance during the day, improve your sleep habits.

Do's

WEEK OF _____

GOALS FOR THIS WEEK
① _____
② _____
③ _____

MONDAY ① ② ③	**TUESDAY** ① ② ③

WEDNESDAY ① ② ③	**THURSDAY** ① ② ③

FRIDAY ① ② ③	**SATURDAY** ① ② ③

SUNDAY ① ② ③

A clever person solves a problem. A wise person avoids it.
— Albert Einstein

Doodles & Dreams

Feel Good Tip #3 To knock stress down to size, think balance.

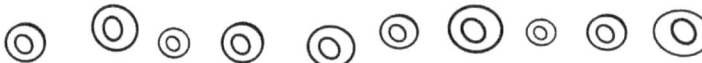

Do'y

WEEK OF _____

GOALS FOR THIS WEEK
① _____
② _____
③ _____

MONDAY   ① ② ③

TUESDAY   ① ② ③

WEDNESDAY   ① ② ③

THURSDAY   ① ② ③

FRIDAY   ① ② ③

SATURDAY   ① ② ③

SUNDAY   ① ② ③

Do what you feel in your heart to be right—for you'll be criticized anyway.
—Eleanor Roosevelt

Doodles & Dreams

FEEL GOOD Tip #4 To relax, make time to reflect.

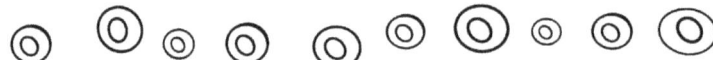

Do'y

WEEK OF _____

GOALS FOR THIS WEEK
① _____
② _____
③ _____

MONDAY ① ② ③

TUESDAY ① ② ③

WEDNESDAY ① ② ③

THURSDAY ① ② ③

FRIDAY ① ② ③

SATURDAY ① ② ③

SUNDAY ① ② ③

We are what we repeatedly do. Excellence, then, is not an act, but a habit.
— Aristotle

Doodles & Dreams

FEEL GOOD Tip #5 To stay in the stress-free zone, say hello to yoga.

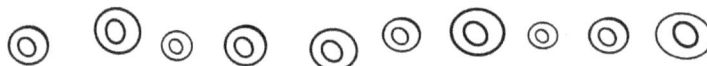

Do's

WEEK OF _____

GOALS FOR THIS WEEK
① _____
② _____
③ _____

MONDAY ① ② ③	**TUESDAY** ① ② ③

WEDNESDAY ① ② ③	**THURSDAY** ① ② ③

FRIDAY ① ② ③	**SATURDAY** ① ② ③

SUNDAY ① ② ③

If you want to go quickly, go alone, if you want to go far, go together.
—African proverb

Doodles & Dreams

FEEL GOOD Tip #6 To help banish test anxiety, get enough vitamin C.

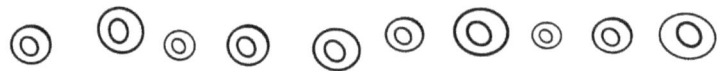

Do's

WEEK OF _____

GOALS FOR THIS WEEK
① _____
② _____
③ _____

MONDAY ① ② ③	**TUESDAY** ① ② ③

WEDNESDAY ① ② ③	**THURSDAY** ① ② ③

FRIDAY ① ② ③	**SATURDAY** ① ② ③

SUNDAY ① ② ③

I hear and I forget. I see and I remember. I do and I understand.
—*Confucius*

Doodles & Dreams

FEEL GOOD Tip #7 To fuel your body (and brain), fill your plate with veggies and fruits.

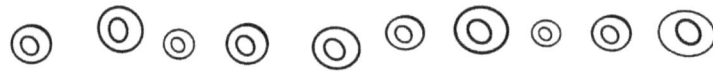

Do'y

WEEK OF _____

GOALS FOR THIS WEEK
① _____
② _____
③ _____

MONDAY ① ② ③	**TUESDAY** ① ② ③

WEDNESDAY ① ② ③	**THURSDAY** ① ② ③

FRIDAY ① ② ③	**SATURDAY** ① ② ③

SUNDAY ① ② ③

Whatever you can do, or dream you can do, begin it. Boldness has genius, power and magic in it. Begin it now.
—Johann Wolfgang von Goethe

Doodles & Dreams

FEEL GOOD Tip #8 To get more from plant foods, eat a variety in a rainbow of colors.

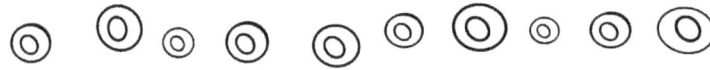

Do's

WEEK OF _____

GOALS FOR THIS WEEK
① _____
② _____
③ _____

MONDAY   ① ② ③

TUESDAY   ① ② ③

WEDNESDAY   ① ② ③

THURSDAY   ① ② ③

FRIDAY   ① ② ③

SATURDAY   ① ② ③

SUNDAY   ① ② ③

A good laugh and a long sleep are the best cures in the doctor's book.
— Irish proverb

Doodles & Dreams

Feel Good Tip #9 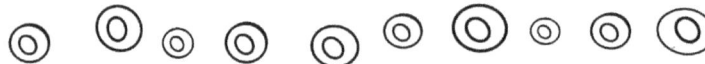 For a phytonutrient payload, eat more salads.

Day

WEEK OF _____

GOALS FOR THIS WEEK
① _____
② _____
③ _____

MONDAY ① ② ③

TUESDAY ① ② ③

WEDNESDAY ① ② ③

THURSDAY ① ② ③

FRIDAY ① ② ③

SATURDAY ① ② ③

SUNDAY ① ② ③

*We first make our habits,
then our habits make us.*
—John Dryden

Doodles & Dreams

FEEL GOOD Tip #10 To detoxify and fortify your health, eat more cruciferous veggies.

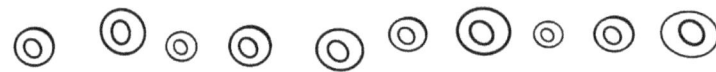

Do's

WEEK OF _____

GOALS FOR THIS WEEK
① _____
② _____
③ _____

MONDAY ① ② ③	TUESDAY ① ② ③

WEDNESDAY ① ② ③	THURSDAY ① ② ③

FRIDAY ① ② ③	SATURDAY ① ② ③

SUNDAY ① ② ③	
	Absorb what is useful. Discard what is not. Add what is uniquely your own. —Bruce Lee

Doodles & Dreams

FEEL GOOD Tip #11 To brighten up a meal, add a colorful grain.

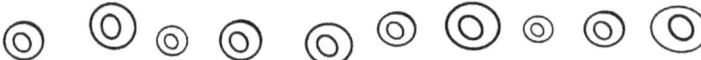

Do'y

Week of _____

Goals for this week
① _____
② _____
③ _____

Monday ① ② ③	**Tuesday** ① ② ③

Wednesday ① ② ③	**Thursday** ① ② ③

Friday ① ② ③	**Saturday** ① ② ③

Sunday ① ② ③

Be kind whenever possible.
It is always possible.
　　　　　—Dalai Lama

Doodles & Dreams

FEEL GOOD
Tip #12 To get more from life, take time to taste.

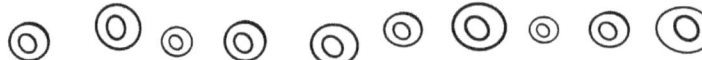

Do'y

WEEK OF _____

GOALS FOR THIS WEEK
① _____
② _____
③ _____

MONDAY ① ② ③	**TUESDAY** ① ② ③

WEDNESDAY ① ② ③	**THURSDAY** ① ② ③

FRIDAY ① ② ③	**SATURDAY** ① ② ③

SUNDAY ① ② ③	
	Always do your best. What you plant now, you will harvest later. —Og Mandino

Doodles & Dreams

FEEL GOOD Tip #13 To encourage a friend, send an inspiring text message.

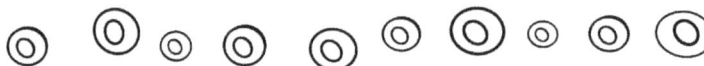

Do's

WEEK OF _____

GOALS FOR THIS WEEK
① _____
② _____
③ _____

MONDAY ① ② ③	**TUESDAY** ① ② ③

WEDNESDAY ① ② ③	**THURSDAY** ① ② ③

FRIDAY ① ② ③	**SATURDAY** ① ② ③

SUNDAY ① ② ③	
	Don't carry your mistakes around. Instead place them under your feet to use as stepping stones. 　　　　—Anonymous

Doodles & Dreams

FEEL GOOD Tip #14 For better heart health, volunteer to help others.

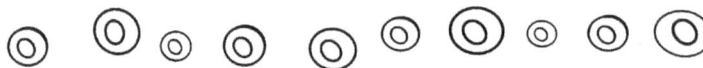

Do's

WEEK OF _____

GOALS FOR THIS WEEK
① _____
② _____
③ _____

MONDAY ① ② ③

TUESDAY ① ② ③

WEDNESDAY ① ② ③

THURSDAY ① ② ③

FRIDAY ① ② ③

SATURDAY ① ② ③

SUNDAY ① ② ③

*Wherever you go,
go with all your heart.*
—*Confucius*

Doodles & Dreams

FEEL GOOD
Tip #15
For a happier day, move more.

Do's

WEEK OF _____

GOALS FOR THIS WEEK
① _____
② _____
③ _____

MONDAY ① ② ③

TUESDAY ① ② ③

WEDNESDAY ① ② ③

THURSDAY ① ② ③

FRIDAY ① ② ③

SATURDAY ① ② ③

SUNDAY ① ② ③

Earth laughs in flowers.
— *Ralph Waldo Emerson*

Doodles & Dreams

LOOK GOOD Tip #1 To put your best face forward, eat more carotenoid-rich veggies and fruits.

Do's

WEEK OF _____

GOALS FOR THIS WEEK
① _____
② _____
③ _____

MONDAY ① ② ③	**TUESDAY** ① ② ③

WEDNESDAY ① ② ③	**THURSDAY** ① ② ③

FRIDAY ① ② ③	**SATURDAY** ① ② ③

SUNDAY ① ② ③

If I cannot do great things, I can do small things in a great way.
—Martin Luther King

Doodles & Dreams

LOOK GOOD Tip #2 For a clear skin routine that really works, fill your plate with low-GI foods.

Do's

WEEK OF _____

GOALS FOR THIS WEEK
① _____
② _____
③ _____

MONDAY ① ② ③	**TUESDAY** ① ② ③
WEDNESDAY ① ② ③	**THURSDAY** ① ② ③
FRIDAY ① ② ③	**SATURDAY** ① ② ③
SUNDAY ① ② ③	

*Every smile makes
you a day younger.*
—Chinese proverb

Doodles & Dreams

LOOK GOOD Tip #3 To soothe dry, itchy winter skin, get enough vitamin D.

Do's

WEEK OF _____

GOALS FOR THIS WEEK
① _____
② _____
③ _____

MONDAY ① ② ③	**TUESDAY** ① ② ③

WEDNESDAY ① ② ③	**THURSDAY** ① ② ③

FRIDAY ① ② ③	**SATURDAY** ① ② ③

SUNDAY ① ② ③

All truly great thoughts are conceived while walking.
—*Friedrich Nietzsche*

Doodles & Dreams

LOOK GOOD Tip #4 To control acne severity, consume more skin-friendly fats.

Do's

Week of _____

Goals for this week
① _____
② _____
③ _____

Monday ① ② ③

Tuesday ① ② ③

Wednesday ① ② ③

Thursday ① ② ③

Friday ① ② ③

Saturday ① ② ③

Sunday ① ② ③

Every tooth in a man's head is more valuable than a diamond.
—Miguel de Cervantes

Doodles & Dreams

LOOK GOOD
Tip #5 To fight acne, turn to the power of vitamin A.

Do's

WEEK OF _____

GOALS FOR THIS WEEK
① _____
② _____
③ _____

MONDAY ① ② ③	**TUESDAY** ① ② ③

WEDNESDAY ① ② ③	**THURSDAY** ① ② ③

FRIDAY ① ② ③	**SATURDAY** ① ② ③

SUNDAY ① ② ③

Honest disagreement is often a good sign of progress.
—*Mahatma Gandhi*

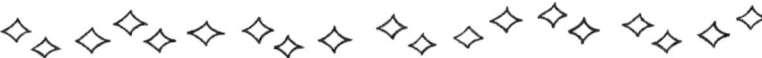

Doodles & Dreams

LOOK GOOD Tip #6 To smile bright, fine-tune your food choices and eating habits.

Do's

WEEK OF _____

GOALS FOR THIS WEEK
① _____
② _____
③ _____

MONDAY ① ② ③

TUESDAY ① ② ③

WEDNESDAY ① ② ③

THURSDAY ① ② ③

FRIDAY ① ② ③

SATURDAY ① ② ③

SUNDAY ① ② ③

Everyone must take time to sit and watch the leaves turn.
—Elizabeth Lawrence

Doodles & Dreams

LOOK GOOD Tip #7 To protect your dazzling smile, pick the right kind of gum.

Do'y

WEEK OF _____

GOALS FOR THIS WEEK
① _____
② _____
③ _____

MONDAY ① ② ③	**TUESDAY** ① ② ③

WEDNESDAY ① ② ③	**THURSDAY** ① ② ③

FRIDAY ① ② ③	**SATURDAY** ① ② ③

SUNDAY ① ② ③

Happiness held is the seed.
Happiness shared is the flower.
—*John Harrigan*

Doodles & Dreams

LOOK GOOD Tip #8 To protect your pearly whites, lighten up on sports and energy drinks.

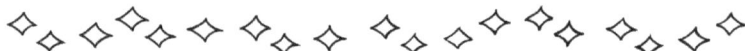

Doʒy

WEEK OF _____

GOALS FOR THIS WEEK
① _____
② _____
③ _____

MONDAY ① ② ③	**TUESDAY** ① ② ③
WEDNESDAY ① ② ③	**THURSDAY** ① ② ③
FRIDAY ① ② ③	**SATURDAY** ① ② ③
SUNDAY ① ② ③	

I took a walk in the woods and came out taller than the trees.
—Henry David Thoreau

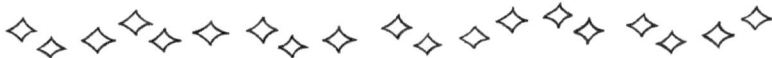

Doodles & Dreams

LOOK GOOD Tip #9 To avoid eye strain, fill your plate with lutein-rich foods and take blinking breaks.

Do's

WEEK OF _____

GOALS FOR THIS WEEK
① _____
② _____
③ _____

MONDAY ① ② ③

TUESDAY ① ② ③

WEDNESDAY ① ② ③

THURSDAY ① ② ③

FRIDAY ① ② ③

SATURDAY ① ② ③

SUNDAY ① ② ③

*Everything has beauty,
but not everyone sees it.*
—Confucius

Doodles & Dreams

LOOK GOOD Tip #10 To unleash your growth potential, get enough calcium.

Do'y

WEEK OF _____

GOALS FOR THIS WEEK
① _____
② _____
③ _____

| **MONDAY** ① ② ③ | **TUESDAY** ① ② ③ |

| **WEDNESDAY** ① ② ③ | **THURSDAY** ① ② ③ |

| **FRIDAY** ① ② ③ | **SATURDAY** ① ② ③ |

SUNDAY ① ② ③

If you can't explain it simply, you don't understand it well enough.
—Albert Einstein

Doodles & Dreams

**LOOK GOOD
Tip #11** For stronger bones, know all the nutrients that matter.

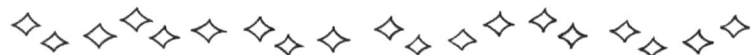

Do'y

WEEK OF _____

GOALS FOR THIS WEEK
① _____
② _____
③ _____

MONDAY ① ② ③	TUESDAY ① ② ③
WEDNESDAY ① ② ③	THURSDAY ① ② ③
FRIDAY ① ② ③	SATURDAY ① ② ③
SUNDAY ① ② ③	

*Time is a created thing.
To say 'I don't have
time,' is like saying,
'I don't want to.'*
—Lao Tzu

Doodles & Dreams

LOOK GOOD
Tip #12 To instantly look better, stand tall.

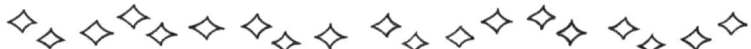

Do's

WEEK OF _____

GOALS FOR THIS WEEK
① _____
② _____
③ _____

MONDAY ① ② ③

TUESDAY ① ② ③

WEDNESDAY ① ② ③

THURSDAY ① ② ③

FRIDAY ① ② ③

SATURDAY ① ② ③

SUNDAY ① ② ③

Make each day your masterpiece.
—John Wooden

Doodles & Dreams

LOOK GOOD
Tip #13 For muscle building, eat enough protein.

Do'y

WEEK OF _____

GOALS FOR THIS WEEK
① _____
② _____
③ _____

MONDAY ① ② ③	**TUESDAY** ① ② ③

WEDNESDAY ① ② ③	**THURSDAY** ① ② ③

FRIDAY ① ② ③	**SATURDAY** ① ② ③

SUNDAY ① ② ③

It is our attitude at the beginning of a difficult task which, more than anything else, will affect its successful outcome.
—Williams James

Doodles & Dreams

Look Good Tip #14 For muscle building, choose protein foods rich in leucine.

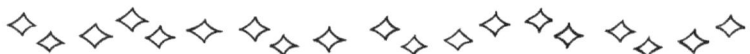

Do's

WEEK OF _____

GOALS FOR THIS WEEK
① _____
② _____
③ _____

MONDAY ① ② ③	**TUESDAY** ① ② ③

WEDNESDAY ① ② ③	**THURSDAY** ① ② ③

FRIDAY ① ② ③	**SATURDAY** ① ② ③

SUNDAY ① ② ③

Life is not measured by the number of breaths we take, but by the moments that take our breath away.
—Maya Angelou

Doodles & Dreams

Look Good Tip #15 For muscle building, eat protein foods at the right time.

Do'y

Week of _____

Goals for this week
① _____
② _____
③ _____

Monday ① ② ③	**Tuesday** ① ② ③

Wednesday ① ② ③	**Thursday** ① ② ③

Friday ① ② ③	**Saturday** ① ② ③

Sunday ① ② ③

Nothing great was ever achieved without enthusiasm.
—Ralph Waldo Emerson

Doodles & Dreams

SUCCESS Tip #1 — To be your best, fill your plate for performance.

Do'y

Week of _____

Goals for this week
① _____
② _____
③ _____

Monday ① ② ③	**Tuesday** ① ② ③

Wednesday ① ② ③	**Thursday** ① ② ③

Friday ① ② ③	**Saturday** ① ② ③

Sunday ① ② ③

One kind word can warm three winter months.
—*Japanese proverb*

Doodles & Dreams

SUCCESS Tip #2 To feel full and satisfied, eat enough fiber.

Do'y

WEEK OF _____

GOALS FOR THIS WEEK
① _____
② _____
③ _____

MONDAY ① ② ③	**TUESDAY** ① ② ③
WEDNESDAY ① ② ③	**THURSDAY** ① ② ③
FRIDAY ① ② ③	**SATURDAY** ① ② ③
SUNDAY ① ② ③	

Pull up a chair. Take a taste. Come join us. Life is so endlessly delicious.
— Ruth Reichi

Doodles & Dreams

Success Tip #3 To make sure you're fully hydrated, take a look at your pee.

Do's

WEEK OF _____

GOALS FOR THIS WEEK
① _____
② _____
③ _____

MONDAY ① ② ③	**TUESDAY** ① ② ③
WEDNESDAY ① ② ③	**THURSDAY** ① ② ③
FRIDAY ① ② ③	**SATURDAY** ① ② ③
SUNDAY ① ② ③	

Our lives are ultimately a reflection of the choices we make each day.
— *Anonymous*

Doodles & Dreams

SUCCESS Tip #4 — To control inflammation, say goodbye to added sugars.

Do's

WEEK OF _____

GOALS FOR THIS WEEK
① _____
② _____
③ _____

MONDAY ① ② ③	**TUESDAY** ① ② ③
WEDNESDAY ① ② ③	**THURSDAY** ① ② ③
FRIDAY ① ② ③	**SATURDAY** ① ② ③
SUNDAY ① ② ③	

Creativity is intelligence having fun.
　　—*Albert Einstein*

Doodles & Dreams

SUCCESS Tip #5 To be ready for early morning zero periods, prepare the no-brainer way.

Do's

WEEK OF _____

GOALS FOR THIS WEEK
① _____
② _____
③ _____

MONDAY ① ② ③	**TUESDAY** ① ② ③

WEDNESDAY ① ② ③	**THURSDAY** ① ② ③

FRIDAY ① ② ③	**SATURDAY** ① ② ③

SUNDAY ① ② ③

Short cuts make long delays.
—JRR Tolkien

Doodles & Dreams

SUCCESS Tip #6 For benefits that last all day, eat a high-protein breakfast.

Do's

WEEK OF _____

GOALS FOR THIS WEEK
① _____
② _____
③ _____

MONDAY ① ② ③

TUESDAY ① ② ③

WEDNESDAY ① ② ③

THURSDAY ① ② ③

FRIDAY ① ② ③

SATURDAY ① ② ③

SUNDAY ① ② ③

Overcome the notion that we must be regular…it robs you of the chance to be extraordinary.
— Uta Hagan

Doodles & Dreams

SUCCESS Tip #7 To banish caffeine jitters, find your Goldilocks balance.

Do's

WEEK OF _____

GOALS FOR THIS WEEK
① _____
② _____
③ _____

MONDAY ① ② ③	**TUESDAY** ① ② ③

WEDNESDAY ① ② ③	**THURSDAY** ① ② ③

FRIDAY ① ② ③	**SATURDAY** ① ② ③

SUNDAY ① ② ③

The best way to cheer yourself up is to cheer someone else up.
—Mark Twain

Doodles & Dreams

SUCCESS
Tip #8 For better test scores, fine-tune how you eat.

Do'y

WEEK OF _____

GOALS FOR THIS WEEK
① _____
② _____
③ _____

MONDAY ① ② ③	**TUESDAY** ① ② ③

WEDNESDAY ① ② ③	**THURSDAY** ① ② ③

FRIDAY ① ② ③	**SATURDAY** ① ② ③

SUNDAY ① ② ③

I cannot teach anybody anything, I can only make them think.
—Socrates

Doodles & Dreams

SUCCESS Tip #9 For strong immunity, start with what you eat.

Do's

WEEK OF _____

GOALS FOR THIS WEEK
① _____
② _____
③ _____

MONDAY ① ② ③

TUESDAY ① ② ③

WEDNESDAY ① ② ③

THURSDAY ① ② ③

FRIDAY ① ② ③

SATURDAY ① ② ③

SUNDAY ① ② ③

The only real mistake is the one from which we learn nothing.
—*John Powell*

Doodles & Dreams

SUCCESS Tip #10 To fully enjoy your winter adventures, fortify your immune health.

Do's

WEEK OF _____

GOALS FOR THIS WEEK
① _____
② _____
③ _____

MONDAY ① ② ③	**TUESDAY** ① ② ③
WEDNESDAY ① ② ③	**THURSDAY** ① ② ③
FRIDAY ① ② ③	**SATURDAY** ① ② ③
SUNDAY ① ② ③	

We make a living by what we get, but we make a life by what we give.
—*Winston Churchill*

Doodles & Dreams

SUCCESS Tip #11 To be healthier, happier and more successful, try the mealtime secret.

Do's

Week of _____

Goals for this week
① _____
② _____
③ _____

Monday ① ② ③	**Tuesday** ① ② ③

Wednesday ① ② ③	**Thursday** ① ② ③

Friday ① ② ③	**Saturday** ① ② ③

Sunday ① ② ③

There is a calmness to a life lived in gratitude, a quiet joy.
—Ralph H. Bloom

Doodles & Dreams

SUCCESS Tip #12 — To lower your pesticide burden, choose cleaner vegetables and fruits.

Do'y

WEEK OF _____

GOALS FOR THIS WEEK
① _____
② _____
③ _____

MONDAY ① ② ③	**TUESDAY** ① ② ③

WEDNESDAY ① ② ③	**THURSDAY** ① ② ③

FRIDAY ① ② ③	**SATURDAY** ① ② ③

SUNDAY ① ② ③

Logic will get you from A to B. Imagination will take you everywhere.
—Albert Einstein

Doodles & Dreams

Success Tip #13 For an easier way to shape new habits, be like bamboo.

Do's

WEEK OF _____

GOALS FOR THIS WEEK
① _____
② _____
③ _____

MONDAY ① ② ③

TUESDAY ① ② ③

WEDNESDAY ① ② ③

THURSDAY ① ② ③

FRIDAY ① ② ③

SATURDAY ① ② ③

SUNDAY ① ② ③

There is more to life than increasing its speed.
—*Mahatma Gandhi*

Doodles & Dreams

SUCCESS Tip #14 Follow your taste buds, and your future self will thank you.

Do's

Week of _____

Goals for this week
① _____
② _____
③ _____

Monday ① ② ③	**Tuesday** ① ② ③

Wednesday ① ② ③	**Thursday** ① ② ③

Friday ① ② ③	**Saturday** ① ② ③

Sunday ① ② ③

We do not inherit the earth from our ancestors, we borrow it from our children.
　—Native American proverb

Doodles & Dreams

Success Tip #15 To fill nutrient gaps, take a daily multivitamin.

Do's

WEEK OF _____

GOALS FOR THIS WEEK
① _____
② _____
③ _____

MONDAY   ① ② ③

TUESDAY   ① ② ③

WEDNESDAY   ① ② ③

THURSDAY   ① ② ③

FRIDAY   ① ② ③

SATURDAY   ① ② ③

SUNDAY   ① ② ③

The mind is everything.
What you think you become.
  —Buddha

Doodles & Dreams

BONUS Tip #1 You can move mountains, but first you need more vegetables (and fruits and whole grains and nuts). See a pattern?

 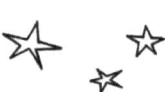

Do'y

WEEK OF _____

GOALS FOR THIS WEEK
① _____
② _____
③ _____

MONDAY ① ② ③

TUESDAY ① ② ③

WEDNESDAY ① ② ③

THURSDAY ① ② ③

FRIDAY ① ② ③

SATURDAY ① ② ③

SUNDAY ① ② ③

There is nothing on this earth more to be prized than true friendship.
—Thomas Acquinas

Doodles & Dreams

BONUS Tip #2 For daily benefits that matter like regularity, satiety and a healthy gut microbiome, eat enough fiber-rich foods.

 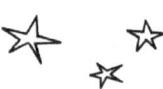

Do'y

WEEK OF _____

GOALS FOR THIS WEEK
① _____
② _____
③ _____

MONDAY ① ② ③	**TUESDAY** ① ② ③

WEDNESDAY ① ② ③	**THURSDAY** ① ② ③

FRIDAY ① ② ③	**SATURDAY** ① ② ③

SUNDAY ① ② ③

You miss 100% of the shots you never take.
—*Wayne Gretzky*

Doodles & Dreams

BONUS Tip #3   Quench your thirst. Drink up to help banish brain fog, fight fatigue, curb your appetite and more. Yes, it's that easy.

 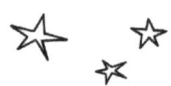

 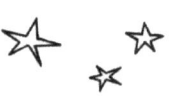

Do's

WEEK OF _____

GOALS FOR THIS WEEK
① _____
② _____
③ _____

MONDAY ① ② ③

TUESDAY ① ② ③

WEDNESDAY ① ② ③

THURSDAY ① ② ③

FRIDAY ① ② ③

SATURDAY ① ② ③

SUNDAY ① ② ③

*Those who wish to sing,
always find a song.*
— Swedish proverb

Doodles & Dreams

BONUS Tip #4 Clear eyes, a sharp mind and a healthy heart. What's not to love? All good stuff made better with omega-3 fats.

 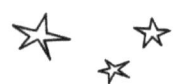

 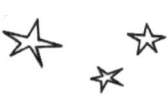

Do's

WEEK OF _____

GOALS FOR THIS WEEK
① _____
② _____
③ _____

MONDAY ① ② ③	**TUESDAY** ① ② ③

WEDNESDAY ① ② ③	**THURSDAY** ① ② ③

FRIDAY ① ② ③	**SATURDAY** ① ② ③

SUNDAY ① ② ③

What sunshine is to flowers, smiles are to humanity.
—Joseph Addison

Doodles & Dreams

BONUS Tip #5 Ready to reclaim your life? It's simple, but not easy. Start with banishing mindless time on your phone.

 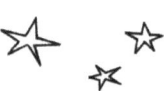

Do'y

WEEK OF _____

GOALS FOR THIS WEEK
① _____
② _____
③ _____

MONDAY ① ② ③	**TUESDAY** ① ② ③
WEDNESDAY ① ② ③	**THURSDAY** ① ② ③
FRIDAY ① ② ③	**SATURDAY** ① ② ③
SUNDAY ① ② ③	

The best way to predict the future is to create it.
—Abraham Lincoln

Doodles & Dreams

BONUS Tip #6 Time your exercise to work for you. You'll feel alert during the day and sleep like a baby at night.

 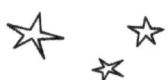

 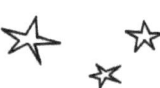

Do'y

WEEK OF _____

GOALS FOR THIS WEEK
① _____
② _____
③ _____

MONDAY ① ② ③

TUESDAY ① ② ③

WEDNESDAY ① ② ③

THURSDAY ① ② ③

FRIDAY ① ② ③

SATURDAY ① ② ③

SUNDAY ① ② ③

We don't rise to the level of our expectations, we fall to the level of our training.
—*Archilochus*

Doodles & Dreams

BONUS
Tip #7
Sleep well, be well. It's almost magical. Wake up from a restful night's sleep, and you're ready to conquer the world.

 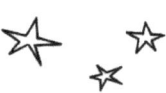

Do's

WEEK OF _____

GOALS FOR THIS WEEK
① _____
② _____
③ _____

MONDAY ① ② ③

TUESDAY ① ② ③

WEDNESDAY ① ② ③

THURSDAY ① ② ③

FRIDAY ① ② ③

SATURDAY ① ② ③

SUNDAY ① ② ③

*With a dream,
anything is possible.*
—Dr. Sam Rehnborg

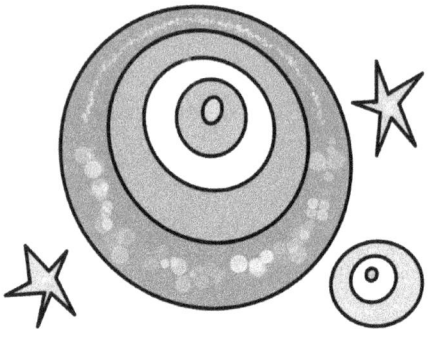

*You're off to Great Places!
Today is your day!
Your mountain is waiting,
So... get on your way!*
— Dr. Seuss

www.ingramcontent.com/pod-product-compliance
Lightning Source LLC
Chambersburg PA
CBHW062102290426
44110CB00022B/2683